HISTAMINE INTOLERANCE FOOD LIST

A Comprehensive Guide and Chart For Low-Histamine Diet including Food to Eat & Avoid

Patricia D. Stotler

Copyright © 2024 by Patricia D. Stotler

Table of Contents

Introduction to Histamine Intolerance

Are You Tired of Feeling Sick After Every Meal? Discover How the Right Foods Can Transform Your Life!

Imagine enjoying a meal without the fear of discomfort, bloating, or severe allergic reactions. What if you could identify precisely what's been causing your symptoms and finally start living the life you deserve? That's the promise of "Histamine Intolerance Food List"—a revolutionary guide that's designed to help you navigate the complex world of histamine intolerance with ease.

The Benefits of Following the "Histamine Intolerance Food List"

This book is more than just a list; it's a comprehensive resource that empowers you to make informed dietary choices. Here are just a few of the benefits you can expect:

- **Relief from Chronic Symptoms:** Learn which foods to avoid to prevent symptoms like headaches, skin irritations, and gastrointestinal discomfort.
- **Increased Energy and Wellbeing:** Discover nutrient-rich, low-histamine foods that boost your energy levels and improve overall health.

- **Customizable Eating Plans:** Tailored strategies that fit into your lifestyle, making it easier to adhere to a low-histamine diet without feeling restricted.

- **Expert Advice and Insight:** Gain knowledge from dietary specialists and the latest scientific research to understand the underlying causes of histamine intolerance.

- **Practical Tips for Everyday Living:** From navigating social situations to understanding food labels, this book provides practical advice that makes low-histamine living seamless and stress-free.

Managing Objections: What Our Book Offers

We understand that changing your diet can be daunting and you might be skeptical about whether this can truly help. Here's how "Histamine Intolerance Food List" addresses common concerns and stands out from the rest:

- **"I've tried everything. How is this different?"**
  - Our book isn't just a diet plan. It's a lifestyle change supported by the latest research. We provide you not only with food lists but also with the science behind histamine intolerance, helping you understand your body better.

- **"Is this just another restrictive diet?"**
  - While it does involve avoiding certain high-histamine foods, our book focuses on a balanced approach to nutrition. We offer a wide range of delicious, safe

alternatives and creative recipes that keep meals exciting and satisfying.

- **"Will I be able to maintain this diet?"**
  - Yes! We provide tools and strategies for adapting to a low-histamine diet, including meal planning guides, tips for eating out, and how to handle social situations without feeling isolated.
- **"What if I don't have time for complicated recipes?"**
  - Our recipes are designed with busy lifestyles in mind. They are simple to prepare, with straightforward ingredients and clear instructions, ensuring that healthy eating fits into your hectic schedule.
- **"How do I know if I'm really histamine intolerant?"**
  - Included in the book is a guide to diagnosis and management, featuring symptoms trackers and advice on when to seek help from a medical professional.

"Histamine Intolerance Food List" is more than just a guide—it's a companion on your journey to better health. This book promises to not only educate you about histamine intolerance but also to provide the support and resources necessary to manage it effectively. Start your journey today and experience the relief and vibrant health you've been missing!

Understanding Histamine

Histamine is a naturally occurring compound that plays a crucial role in the body's immune response to allergens. It is involved in local immune responses as well as regulating physiological function in the gut and acting as a neurotransmitter for the brain, spinal cord, and uterus. Histamine helps to mediate digestion, affect blood vessel permeability, and ensure proper brain function. However, when histamine levels become unbalanced, particularly through the consumption of histamine-rich foods, it can cause a range of symptoms often referred to as histamine intolerance.

Histamine intolerance occurs when there is an accumulation of histamine in the body because the capacity to break it down is overwhelmed or impaired. This is typically due to the dysfunction of the enzyme diamine oxidase (DAO), which is primarily responsible for breaking down ingested histamine. If DAO levels are inadequate, or if one's diet is rich in histamine, the excess histamine can trigger symptoms similar to allergic reactions. These symptoms might include itching, hives, runny nose, headaches, and gastrointestinal discomfort among others.

Certain foods are known to contain high levels of histamine or to trigger the body to release histamine. These include aged cheeses, smoked meats, fermented products like sauerkraut and kombucha, and alcoholic beverages like wine and beer. Additionally, some foods are DAO blockers, which means they inhibit the enzyme responsible for breaking down histamine, exacerbating the symptoms of histamine intolerance.

Avoiding histamine-rich foods is a key strategy for managing histamine intolerance. This involves not only steering clear of foods known to be high in histamine but also those that can trigger histamine release or block DAO activity. The goal of a low-histamine diet is to reduce histamine levels in the body, alleviate symptoms, and support overall health.

Incorporating histamine intolerance management into daily life can significantly improve quality of life for those affected. By understanding which foods to avoid and opting for fresh meat, freshly caught fish, non-citrus fruits, and cooking and eating foods immediately after preparation, individuals can help control their histamine levels and reduce the occurrence of intolerance symptoms. This proactive approach enables those with histamine intolerance to enjoy meals without fear of adverse reactions, leading to a better understanding of their condition and how to manage it effectively.

Causes and Symptoms of Histamine Intolerance

Histamine intolerance occurs when the body accumulates histamine faster than it can break it down, leading to a variety of symptoms that can affect everyday life. The primary cause of this accumulation is often an imbalance between histamine intake and degradation. One common factor is the impaired function of enzymes responsible for breaking down histamine, particularly diamine oxidase (DAO). Genetic factors, gastrointestinal diseases such as leaky gut syndrome, and medications that inhibit DAO activity or enhance histamine release can all contribute to decreased DAO activity or increased histamine levels.

The foods people eat significantly impact histamine levels. High-histamine foods such as aged cheeses, fermented products like sauerkraut and wine, cured meats, and some fish are typical culprits. Additionally, some foods, while not high in histamine themselves, can trigger the release of histamine from other cells in the body or inhibit the activity of enzymes like DAO that break down histamine. These include alcohol, bananas, tomatoes, and chocolate. Consuming these foods can lead to an overload, especially in individuals whose histamine-degrading mechanisms are compromised.

Symptoms of histamine intolerance are diverse and can often mimic other conditions, making diagnosis challenging. They typically include skin irritations such as hives, eczema, or dermatitis, gastrointestinal complaints like diarrhea, nausea, and vomiting, and respiratory issues such as wheezing and nasal congestion. Neurological symptoms such as headaches, migraines, and dizziness are also common. Moreover, some individuals experience low blood pressure or irregular heartbeats. The range and severity of symptoms can vary greatly among individuals, further complicating the recognition and management of histamine intolerance.

Managing histamine intolerance effectively often involves adhering to a low-histamine diet, which means avoiding foods known to be high in histamine or trigger its release. It's essential for individuals to keep a detailed food diary to help identify specific triggers and adjust their diets accordingly. Over time, by carefully selecting and avoiding certain foods, many can significantly reduce their symptoms and improve their quality of life. This strategic approach to diet can be life-changing, offering a return to normalcy and relief from the disruptive and often painful symptoms associated with histamine intolerance.

Diagnosis and Management

Diagnosing histamine intolerance can be challenging because its symptoms often mimic those of other allergies and gastrointestinal disorders. However, the process typically begins with a detailed evaluation of the patient's medical history, followed by an elimination diet and possibly, laboratory tests. During the medical history review, healthcare providers look for a pattern of reaction after consumption of high-histamine foods. If histamine intolerance is suspected, an elimination diet is recommended, where foods known to be high in histamine are strictly avoided for a few weeks. If symptoms improve during this period, high-histamine foods are gradually reintroduced to see if symptoms reappear. This method is often effective in confirming a diagnosis.

Laboratory tests can support the diagnosis, although no single test is definitive for histamine intolerance. Blood tests to measure the levels of histamine and the enzyme diamine oxidase (DAO), which breaks down histamine, can be helpful. Low levels of DAO or elevated levels of histamine may suggest histamine intolerance, but these tests are not widely available and can be inconclusive.

Management of histamine intolerance primarily involves dietary adjustments. Individuals are advised to follow a low-histamine diet, which entails avoiding foods that are naturally high in histamine or that trigger histamine release. These foods include aged cheeses, fermented products like sauerkraut and soy sauce, alcohol, particularly red wine and beer, and processed meats. Fresh foods like freshly cooked meat, non-citrus fruits, and most vegetables are considered safe for those with histamine intolerance.

In addition to dietary changes, management strategies may include the use of supplements such as DAO enzyme supplements, which help break down dietary histamine. Antihistamines can also be effective in managing symptoms, although they do not address the underlying issue of histamine degradation. Regular consultation with a healthcare provider or a dietitian specialized in allergies can provide further personalized guidance and adjustments based on individual responses and nutritional needs.

Long-term management of histamine intolerance also involves addressing any gut health issues since poor gut health can exacerbate the condition. Probiotics and other gut-supporting supplements might be recommended to improve gut flora, which in turn can help in the better breakdown and management of histamine in the body. Lifestyle changes, such as stress reduction techniques, are also advised since stress can trigger or worsen histamine intolerance symptoms.

Overall, the effective management of histamine intolerance requires a comprehensive approach that includes dietary changes, possible supplementation, regular monitoring, and adjustments based on symptom presentation and individual dietary tolerances.

Basics of Histamine Intolerance

What is Histamine?

Histamine is a naturally occurring compound in the human body that plays a crucial role in various physiological functions. It is part of the immune system, helping to fight off pathogens and is also involved in regulating gut function and acting as a neurotransmitter. Histamine is produced by mast cells and basophils, which are types of white blood cells, and is released in response to potential threats like allergens or infections.

When histamine is released, it binds to histamine receptors located throughout the body, triggering different responses depending on the receptor type. For example, histamine is responsible for the classic allergy symptoms of itching, swelling, and runny nose, which occur when it binds to receptors in the respiratory system. It also affects the digestive system, where it stimulates gastric acid secretion, aiding in digestion. Additionally, in the nervous system, histamine functions as a neurotransmitter, contributing to wakefulness and appetite control.

Despite its beneficial roles, histamine can cause issues when it accumulates in high levels. In a healthy individual, histamine is metabolized and broken down efficiently by two main enzymes: diamine oxidase (DAO) and histamine-N-methyltransferase (HNMT). However, in those with histamine intolerance, there may be a deficiency or dysfunction of these enzymes, leading to an excess of histamine in the body. This excess can result from consuming foods high in histamine, which can overwhelm the body's capacity to break it down. Foods such as aged cheeses, fermented products, and alcohol are known to contain high levels of histamine.

When histamine levels rise beyond what the body can handle, it can lead to symptoms such as headaches, skin irritation, gastrointestinal issues, and respiratory problems. The threshold for histamine tolerance varies among individuals, which is why some people can consume high-histamine foods without issues, while others cannot. Histamine intolerance is not an allergy in the conventional sense but rather a sensitivity to dietary and endogenous histamine due to impaired degradation.

Managing histamine intolerance involves following a low-histamine diet, which focuses on avoiding foods that either contain high levels of histamine or trigger its release. This includes certain processed meats, fish, and fermented foods, while emphasizing fresh, minimally processed foods. In addition to dietary adjustments, supplements and medications may help manage symptoms by aiding in histamine breakdown or blocking its effects on receptors. Understanding the role and functions of histamine is key to effectively managing histamine intolerance, as it helps guide appropriate dietary and lifestyle choices for affected individuals.

Diagnosis of Histamine Intolerance

Diagnosing histamine intolerance can be challenging due to its varied symptoms, which often overlap with other conditions. The process typically involves a combination of clinical evaluation, dietary experimentation, and sometimes laboratory testing.

Clinical evaluation starts with a detailed medical history, where a healthcare provider will review the patient's symptoms and any potential triggers. Symptoms commonly associated with histamine intolerance include headaches, flushing, nasal congestion, gastrointestinal issues, and skin reactions. Since these symptoms are non-specific, healthcare providers also consider the patient's dietary habits and any correlations between symptom flare-ups and the consumption of certain foods.

Dietary experimentation often follows, utilizing an elimination diet to identify potential triggers. In this approach, individuals remove high-histamine foods from their diet for several weeks and then gradually reintroduce them. Improvement in symptoms during the elimination phase and their recurrence upon reintroduction strongly suggest histamine intolerance. Common high-histamine foods include aged cheeses, processed meats, fermented products, and alcohol, while low-histamine alternatives might include fresh meats, certain vegetables, and non-citrus fruits.

Laboratory testing, while not definitive, can support the diagnosis of histamine intolerance. Blood tests may measure histamine levels or the activity of diamine oxidase (DAO), the enzyme responsible for breaking down histamine. Low DAO levels or high histamine levels might indicate histamine intolerance, although these tests are not routinely used due to their inconsistent accuracy and availability.

It's important to differentiate histamine intolerance from other conditions with similar symptoms, such as food allergies, irritable bowel syndrome, or mast cell activation syndrome. Healthcare providers may use differential diagnosis techniques, including allergy testing or assessments for other gastrointestinal disorders, to rule out these possibilities.

In addition to these diagnostic steps, some healthcare providers may use a histamine challenge test, where the patient consumes a high-histamine food and is monitored for symptoms. However, this test can be risky due to the potential for severe reactions, so it is not commonly performed.

Once histamine intolerance is diagnosed, the focus shifts to management, which primarily involves dietary modifications. By following a low-histamine diet and avoiding known triggers, most individuals with histamine intolerance can effectively manage their symptoms.

Principles of a Low-Histamine Diet

The Role of Diet in Managing Symptoms

In managing histamine intolerance, diet plays a crucial role in mitigating symptoms and improving overall well-being. The principles of a low-histamine diet revolve around minimizing the intake of foods that are high in histamine or that trigger its release in the body. This dietary approach aims to prevent the accumulation of excess histamine, which can lead to various symptoms such as headaches, gastrointestinal discomfort, skin rashes, and respiratory issues.

The first principle of a low-histamine diet is to identify and avoid foods that contain high levels of histamine. These foods include aged and fermented products, such as aged cheeses, processed meats, and alcoholic beverages, particularly red wine and beer. Fermented foods like sauerkraut, kimchi, and soy sauce are also high in histamine and should be avoided. Fresh meats and seafood should be consumed soon after purchase, as histamine levels increase as these foods age.

Another key aspect of the diet is avoiding foods that stimulate the release of histamine. Certain foods, while not necessarily high in histamine, can trigger the body to release histamine, exacerbating symptoms. These include foods like citrus fruits, tomatoes, eggplants, and certain spices. Additionally, some foods, such as alcohol and energy drinks, inhibit the enzyme diamine oxidase (DAO), which is responsible for breaking down histamine. Consuming these inhibitors can lead to higher histamine levels and should therefore be limited.

It's also important to focus on foods that are low in histamine and unlikely to cause reactions. These include fresh, non-processed meats, most fresh vegetables, except for those that stimulate histamine release, and certain fresh fruits. Dairy alternatives like coconut milk and rice milk are generally well-tolerated, as are grains like rice and oats. Incorporating these foods into the diet can help provide necessary nutrients while minimizing the risk of histamine accumulation.

Maintaining a balanced and varied diet is essential when managing histamine intolerance. While it's important to avoid high-histamine foods, individuals should also ensure they are getting adequate nutrition. This might involve working with a dietitian to develop meal plans that meet nutritional needs while staying within the parameters of a low-histamine diet.

Monitoring and tracking symptoms are also vital components of managing histamine intolerance through diet. Keeping a food diary helps identify potential triggers and tailor the diet to individual tolerances. This personalized approach is key because the severity of histamine intolerance varies among individuals, and what may be tolerated by one person could cause severe reactions in another.

In conclusion, the role of diet in managing symptoms of histamine intolerance is central to controlling and reducing adverse reactions. By focusing on fresh, low-histamine foods, avoiding triggers, and maintaining a balanced diet, individuals can effectively manage their symptoms and improve their quality of life.

Basic Guidelines for a Low-Histamine Diet

A low-histamine diet focuses on reducing the intake of foods that are either high in histamine or trigger its release within the body. The goal of this dietary approach is to minimize histamine-related symptoms such as headaches, skin rashes, digestive issues, and more. To adhere to a low-histamine diet, certain fundamental principles should be followed.

First and foremost, it's important to identify and avoid foods that are naturally high in histamine. These include aged cheeses, processed meats, fermented foods like sauerkraut and soy sauce, alcoholic beverages, especially red wine and beer, and certain fish like tuna and mackerel. These foods have high histamine levels because of the processes they undergo during preparation and storage.

Additionally, foods that are known to stimulate the release of histamine or block the activity of diamine oxidase (DAO), an enzyme crucial for breaking down histamine, should also be avoided. These include certain fruits like bananas, strawberries, and tomatoes, as well as foods like chocolate, nuts, and shellfish.

Freshness is key when following a low-histamine diet. Histamine levels increase as food ages or undergoes prolonged storage, so consuming fresh, unprocessed foods is crucial. Fresh meats and fish should be prepared and consumed quickly after purchase, while leftovers should be minimized or stored immediately in the freezer to prevent histamine buildup.

It's also important to focus on foods that are considered safe for those with histamine intolerance. Fresh, unprocessed meats, most fresh vegetables, and non-citrus fruits like apples and pears are generally well-tolerated. Rice, pasta, and other grains are also typically low in histamine, making them safe staples for meals.

For drinks, water, herbal teas, and freshly squeezed juices from low-histamine fruits are good options. Alcoholic beverages should be avoided due to their high histamine content and their tendency to inhibit DAO activity.

Cooking methods also matter on a low-histamine diet. Slow-cooking methods that involve prolonged cooking times, such as stewing, can increase histamine levels in foods. Quick-cooking methods like grilling, steaming, or sautéing are preferable.

Individuals should also pay attention to their body's unique responses to different foods, as histamine intolerance can vary widely. Keeping a food diary to track symptoms and identify potential triggers can be incredibly helpful for personalized dietary adjustments.

Finally, planning meals in advance and being mindful of potential sources of hidden histamine in processed foods or restaurant dishes is crucial. Reading labels carefully and communicating dietary needs when dining out can help prevent accidental histamine exposure.

Following these basic guidelines for a low-histamine diet can significantly alleviate symptoms for those with histamine intolerance, contributing to improved health and quality of life.

Comprehensive List of Foods to Avoid

Meats and Fish

Food	Description	Reason to Avoid
Tuna	Saltwater fish, high histamine content	Contains high levels of histamine, especially when canned
Mackerel	Fatty fish, high histamine content	Highly prone to histamine formation after catching
Anchovies	Small fish, often canned	Highly fermented, containing excessive histamine
Sardines	Small oily fish	High in histamine, especially when canned
Salami	Cured sausage, fermented	Fermented, resulting in high histamine levels
Pepperoni	Spiced sausage, cured	Contains histamine and other biogenic amines
Smoked Salmon	Smoked fish, preserved	Smoking process increases histamine

Food	Description	Reason to Avoid
Corned Beef	Salt-cured beef	Curing process elevates histamine content
Bacon	Cured pork, smoked	Curing and smoking raise histamine levels
Ham	Cured pork meat	Cured meat, typically high in histamine
Hot Dogs	Processed meat, mixed ingredients	Contains additives and preservatives that elevate histamine
Bologna	Processed sausage, mixed meats	Contains high levels of histamine and additives
Chicken Liver	Organ meat, nutrient-rich	Organs generally contain higher histamine levels
Beef Jerky	Dried beef, seasoned	Drying and seasoning processes increase histamine
Dried Fish	Dehydrated fish, preserved	Dehydrating fish raises histamine to high levels

These meats and fish contain high levels of histamine or are prone to developing high histamine levels during processing or storage, making them problematic for individuals with histamine intolerance.

Dairy Products

Dairy Product	Reason to Avoid	Additional Notes
Aged Cheeses	High in histamine due to aging process	Cheddar, Swiss, Parmesan, and Blue Cheese are examples
Yogurt	Contains live bacteria which can produce histamine	Both regular and Greek yogurt should be avoided
Sour Cream	Fermentation process increases histamine levels	Look for dairy-free alternatives
Buttermilk	Fermentation process increases histamine levels	Often used in baking; substitute with non-dairy milk + vinegar
Cottage Cheese	Fermentation process increases histamine levels	Choose dairy-free cottage cheese or other alternatives
Cream Cheese	Fermentation process increases histamine levels	Often used in spreads and dips; opt for dairy-free versions

Dairy Product	Reason to Avoid	Additional Notes
Ricotta Cheese	Naturally high in histamine	Used in Italian dishes; try vegan ricotta as an alternative
Blue Cheese	High in histamine due to mold growth	Avoid all blue-veined cheeses like Gorgonzola and Roquefort
Brie	High in histamine due to mold growth	Soft cheeses should generally be avoided
Camembert	High in histamine due to mold growth	Soft cheeses like Camembert should be substituted with vegan options
Goat Cheese	Naturally high in histamine	Aged goat cheese especially problematic; fresh might be better
Kefir	Fermented, contains live bacteria	Avoid all fermented dairy drinks like kefir
Ice Cream	Contains dairy and often other histamine triggers	Look for dairy-free, low-histamine ice cream alternatives

Dairy Product	Reason to Avoid	Additional Notes
Milk	High in lactose and can inhibit DAO enzyme	Try non-dairy milk alternatives like almond or coconut milk
Whipped Cream	Contains lactose and is often sweetened	Opt for coconut whipped cream or other dairy-free options

Dairy products are often problematic for individuals with histamine intolerance because they can either naturally contain high levels of histamine or interfere with the body's ability to break down histamine.

Aged Cheeses such as Cheddar, Swiss, and Blue Cheese, along with other aged or moldy cheeses like Brie and Camembert, are particularly high in histamine due to their aging processes and mold growth.

Fermented dairy products like Yogurt, Sour Cream, and Kefir contain live bacteria that produce histamine during fermentation. **Cottage Cheese** and **Ricotta Cheese** should also be avoided, as they undergo similar processes.

Cream Cheese and **Whipped Cream** can contain additives or other ingredients that exacerbate symptoms, while **Ice Cream** typically contains dairy and other potential triggers.

Milk and other lactose-containing products can inhibit the DAO enzyme, which is crucial for histamine breakdown.

Avoiding these dairy products and opting for dairy-free alternatives can significantly alleviate symptoms for those with histamine intolerance. Additionally, keeping an eye on ingredient labels and experimenting with non-dairy substitutes can help individuals maintain a balanced and enjoyable diet.

Vegetables and Fruits

Vegetable/Fruit	Why Avoid	Typical Use
Tomatoes	High in histamine and can trigger symptoms	Used in salads, sauces, and condiments
Spinach	Contains high histamine levels	Eaten fresh in salads or cooked
Eggplant	Contains high histamine levels	Used in various dishes, often baked
Avocado	Known histamine liberator	Used in salads, dips, and on toast
Strawberries	High in histamine and a common trigger	Consumed fresh, in desserts, or as a snack
Citrus Fruits	Trigger histamine release	Consumed fresh or used for juice
Bananas	Known histamine liberator	Consumed fresh or used in baking
Pineapple	Contains high histamine levels	Eaten fresh or used in desserts
Plums	Known histamine liberator	Eaten fresh or used in baking

Vegetable/Fruit	Why Avoid	Typical Use
Papaya	Known histamine liberator	Eaten fresh or used in smoothies
Peppers	Contains high histamine levels	Used in salads, stir-fries, and sauces
Sauerkraut (Cabbage)	Contains high histamine levels due to fermentation	Used as a side or topping
Olives	High in histamine and a common trigger	Consumed as a snack or in salads
Pickles	Contains high histamine levels due to fermentation	Eaten as a snack or side
Cherries	Known histamine liberator	Eaten fresh or used in desserts

Individuals with histamine intolerance should avoid these vegetables and fruits due to their potential to either contain high levels of histamine, act as histamine liberators, or inhibit diamine oxidase (DAO) activity. This dietary caution can help prevent or minimize histamine-related symptoms such as headaches, digestive issues, skin rashes, and more, thus enhancing overall well-being.

Beverages and Alcoholic Drinks

Beverage/Alcoholic Drink	Reason to Avoid
Red Wine	Contains high levels of histamine due to the fermentation process and also inhibits diamine oxidase (DAO) enzyme, which breaks down histamine in the body.
Beer	Contains histamine and tyramine, which can trigger symptoms; also contains yeast, a common trigger for those with histamine intolerance.
Champagne	Similar to other wines, champagne contains high levels of histamine and can inhibit DAO activity.
White Wine	Although lower in histamine than red wine, white wine can still cause reactions due to sulfites and other additives that affect histamine degradation.
Flavored Vodka	Flavored vodkas often contain artificial additives and flavorings that can exacerbate histamine intolerance

Beverage/Alcoholic Drink	Reason to Avoid
	symptoms.
Mixed Cocktails	Cocktails often contain multiple ingredients, including fruit juices and syrups, that are high in histamine or histamine-releasing compounds.
Hard Cider	Hard cider, like beer, is fermented and contains yeast, which can lead to increased histamine levels and symptoms.
Kombucha	This fermented tea drink is high in histamine due to the fermentation process and the presence of yeast and bacteria.
Tonic Water	Tonic water contains quinine, which can release histamine and cause reactions in sensitive individuals.
Fermented Tea	Similar to kombucha, fermented teas are high in histamine due to the fermentation process and the microbial content.

Beverage/Alcoholic Drink	Reason to Avoid
Chocolate Milk	Chocolate contains compounds that can trigger histamine release, while milk can also contribute to histamine issues in some individuals.
Tomato Juice	Tomatoes contain high levels of histamine, and drinking tomato juice can exacerbate symptoms.
Orange Juice	Citrus fruits, including oranges, can release histamine and contribute to symptoms in sensitive individuals.
Apple Cider	Apple cider can ferment and increase histamine levels, and it also contains compounds that can release histamine.
Pre-packaged Smoothies	Pre-packaged smoothies often contain high-histamine fruits, such as bananas and strawberries, and sometimes contain additives that can trigger symptoms.

These beverages and alcoholic drinks either naturally contain high levels of histamine, release histamine within the body, or inhibit the breakdown of histamine, making them problematic for individuals with histamine intolerance. Avoiding these drinks can help mitigate symptoms and improve the overall quality of life for those affected.

Processed Foods and Others

Processed Food	Ingredients/Components	Reason to Avoid
Aged Cheese	Aged milk, salt, enzymes	Contains high levels of histamine due to the aging process.
Cured Meats	Pork/beef, salt, preservatives	High in histamine due to fermentation and preservation processes.
Canned Fish	Fish, salt, sometimes oil	Histamine forms quickly in fish, especially when canned or improperly stored.
Sauerkraut	Fermented cabbage, salt	Fermented foods are high in histamine due to bacterial breakdown.
Soy Sauce	Soybeans, wheat, salt	Fermented condiment, high in histamine due to its

Processed Food	Ingredients/Components	Reason to Avoid
		fermentation process.
Wine Vinegar	Wine, naturally occurring sulfites	Fermented product, often high in histamine and sulfites, which can exacerbate symptoms.
Ketchup	Tomatoes, sugar, vinegar	Contains tomatoes, which are naturally high in histamine and act as histamine liberators.
Beer	Water, barley, hops	Contains yeast and alcohol, both of which increase histamine levels and inhibit DAO enzyme.
Pickles	Cucumbers, vinegar, salt	Fermented, high in histamine due to bacterial breakdown and often contains

Processed Food	Ingredients/Components	Reason to Avoid
		additives.
Processed Yogurt	Milk, live cultures, sugar	Fermented product, high in histamine due to bacterial cultures and often contains added sugar.
Pepperoni	Pork, beef, spices, preservatives	Cured meat, high in histamine due to processing and preservation.
Frozen Pizza	Flour, cheese, tomatoes, toppings	Contains multiple high-histamine ingredients like aged cheese and tomatoes.
Instant Soups	Dehydrated vegetables, salt, preservatives	Often contains additives and ingredients that are histamine liberators, and high salt content.

Processed Food	Ingredients/Components	Reason to Avoid
Bottled Salad Dressings	Oil, vinegar, preservatives	Contains vinegar and preservatives, which are high in histamine or inhibit its breakdown.
Flavored Chips	Potatoes, oils, flavorings	Often contains additives that are histamine liberators and processed oils that inhibit DAO activity.

Each of these processed foods contains ingredients or has undergone processing methods that increase histamine levels or inhibit the enzyme DAO, which helps break down histamine in the body. Avoiding these foods can help individuals with histamine intolerance manage their symptoms more effectively.

Comprehensive List of Foods to Eat

Safe Meats and Protein Sources

Ingredient	Instruction	Nutritional Information	Serving Size	Cooking Time
Chicken Breast	Grill or bake fresh chicken breast with light seasoning	120 calories, 26g protein, 1g fat	3 oz	15-20 mins
Turkey Breast	Roast fresh turkey breast with herbs	125 calories, 27g protein, 1g fat	3 oz	20-25 mins
Rabbit	Slow-cook rabbit with vegetables	120 calories, 22g protein, 4g fat	3 oz	1-1.5 hrs
Lamb	Grill lamb chops with rosemary	250 calories, 25g protein, 15g fat	3 oz	10-12 mins

Ingredient	Instruction	Nutritional Information	Serving Size	Cooking Time
Fresh Pork	Roast lean pork tenderloin with garlic	170 calories, 26g protein, 6g fat	3 oz	25-30 mins
Quail	Roast quail with olive oil and herbs	180 calories, 24g protein, 9g fat	3 oz	20-25 mins
Duck Breast	Pan-sear duck breast with salt and pepper	200 calories, 24g protein, 10g fat	3 oz	10-15 mins
Bison	Grill bison steak with light seasoning	140 calories, 28g protein, 2g fat	3 oz	10-15 mins
Venison	Grill venison medallions with thyme	135 calories, 26g protein, 3g fat	3 oz	10-12 mins
Ostrich	Grill ostrich steak with minimal seasoning	130 calories, 27g protein, 2g fat	3 oz	6-8 mins
Goat	Stew goat with vegetables	150 calories, 25g protein, 5g	3 oz	1.5-2 hrs

Ingredient	Instruction	Nutritional Information	Serving Size	Cooking Time
		fat		
Kangaroo	Grill kangaroo steak with olive oil	110 calories, 26g protein, 1g fat	3 oz	6-8 mins
Pheasant	Roast pheasant with herbs and spices	170 calories, 24g protein, 7g fat	3 oz	20-25 mins
Guinea Fowl	Roast guinea fowl with garlic and herbs	150 calories, 22g protein, 6g fat	3 oz	20-25 mins
Fresh Salmon	Grill fresh salmon fillet with lemon	200 calories, 22g protein, 12g fat	3 oz	10-12 mins

These protein sources are generally considered safe for people with histamine intolerance, provided they are fresh and properly prepared.

Safe Dairy Alternatives

For individuals with histamine intolerance, finding safe alternatives to dairy is crucial as many dairy products are high in histamine or can trigger histamine release.

Dairy Alternative	Key Ingredient(s)	Preparation Instructions	Nutritional Information (per serving)	Serving Size	Cooking Time
1. Almond Milk	Blanched almonds, water	Blend almonds with water, strain through cheesecloth	Low in calories, dairy-free, good source of vitamin E	1 cup (240 ml)	10 minutes
2. Coconut Milk	Coconut meat, water	Blend coconut meat with water, strain	High in medium-chain triglycerides, dairy-free	1 cup (240 ml)	10 minutes
3. Oat Milk	Rolled oats, water	Blend oats with water,	Rich in fiber, low in fat,	1 cup (240	30 minutes

Dairy Alternative	Key Ingredient(s)	Preparation Instructions	Nutritional Information (per serving)	Serving Size	Cooking Time
		strain	dairy-free	ml)	
4. Rice Milk	Brown rice, water	Cook rice, blend with water, strain	Low in protein, high in carbohydrates, dairy-free	1 cup (240 ml)	45 minutes
5. Hemp Milk	Hemp seeds, water	Blend hemp seeds with water, strain	Contains omega-3 and omega-6 fatty acids, dairy-free	1 cup (240 ml)	5 minutes
6. Cashew Milk	Cashews, water	Soak cashews, blend with water, strain	Rich in magnesium and zinc, dairy-free	1 cup (240 ml)	2 hours soaking + 10 minutes blending
7. Soy Milk	Soybeans, water	Soak soybeans,	High in protein, low	1 cup (240	Overnight

Dairy Alternative	Key Ingredient(s)	Preparation Instructions	Nutritional Information (per serving)	Serving Size	Cooking Time
		blend with water, cook, strain	in saturated fat, dairy-free	ml)	soaking + 20 minutes cooking
8. Flax Milk	Flax seeds, water	Blend flax seeds with water, strain	High in omega-3 fatty acids, dairy-free	1 cup (240 ml)	10 minutes
9. Quinoa Milk	Quinoa, water	Cook quinoa, blend with water, strain	Complete protein source, gluten-free, dairy-free	1 cup (240 ml)	30 minutes
10. Macadamia Milk	Macadamia nuts, water	Blend macadamia nuts with water, strain	High in healthy fats, dairy-free	1 cup (240 ml)	10 minutes
11. Pea	Yellow peas,	Blend	High in	1 cup	25

Dairy Alternative	Key Ingredient(s)	Preparation Instructions	Nutritional Information (per serving)	Serving Size	Cooking Time
Milk	water	cooked peas with water, strain	protein, dairy-free, rich in iron	(240 ml)	minutes
12. Hazelnut Milk	Hazelnuts, water	Blend hazelnuts with water, strain	High in vitamin E, dairy-free	1 cup (240 ml)	10 minutes
13. Sesame Milk	Sesame seeds, water	Soak sesame seeds, blend with water, strain	Rich in calcium, dairy-free	1 cup (240 ml)	8 hours soaking + 10 minutes blending
14. Walnut Milk	Walnuts, water	Soak walnuts, blend with water, strain	Rich in omega-3 fatty acids, dairy-free	1 cup (240 ml)	4 hours soaking + 10 minutes blending

Dairy Alternative	Key Ingredient(s)	Preparation Instructions	Nutritional Information (per serving)	Serving Size	Cooking Time
15. Safflower Milk	Safflower seeds, water	Blend safflower seeds with water, strain	Good source of polyunsaturated fats, dairy-free	1 cup (240 ml)	10 minutes

This table offers a variety of dairy-free alternatives that can be made at home with simple ingredients and methods. Each alternative provides different nutritional benefits, making it easier for those with histamine intolerance to maintain a balanced diet while avoiding dairy.

Food	Description	Ingredients	Instructions	Nutritional Information	Serving Size	Cooking Time
Broccoli	Low-histamine vegetable rich in vitamins	Broccoli, olive oil, garlic, salt	Steam or sauté broccoli with olive oil and garlic	Calories: 55, Protein: 3.7g, Carbs: 11.2g, Fiber: 5.1g	1 cup	10 minutes
Cauliflower	Low-histamine, fiber-rich cruciferous veggie	Cauliflower, olive oil, turmeric, salt	Roast cauliflower with olive oil, turmeric, and salt	Calories: 25, Protein: 2g, Carbs: 5g, Fiber: 2g	1 cup	25 minutes

Food	Description	Ingredients	Instructions	Nutritional Information	Serving Size	Cooking Time
Zucchini	Mild, low-histamine veggie	Zucchini, olive oil, pepper, salt	Grill or sauté zucchini with olive oil, pepper, and salt	Calories: 20, Protein: 1.5g, Carbs: 3.5g, Fiber: 1.1g	1 cup	10 minutes
Carrot	Sweet, low-histamine root vegetable	Carrots, honey, olive oil, rosemary	Roast or steam carrots with honey and rosemary	Calories: 50, Protein: 1g, Carbs: 12g, Fiber: 3g	1 cup	15 minutes
Cucumber	Refreshing low-histamine vegetable	Cucumber, olive oil, dill, salt	Slice and mix cucumber with olive oil, dill,	Calories: 16, Protein: 0.6g, Carbs:	1 cup	5 minutes

Food	Description	Ingredients	Instructions	Nutritional Information	Serving Size	Cooking Time
			and salt	3.8g, Fiber: 0.5g		
Green Beans	Low-histamine, fiber-rich veggie	Green beans, butter, garlic, salt	Steam or sauté green beans with butter and garlic	Calories: 44, Protein: 2.4g, Carbs: 10g, Fiber: 3.7g	1 cup	10 minutes
Lettuce	Low-histamine leafy green	Lettuce, olive oil, lemon, salt	Mix lettuce with olive oil, lemon juice, and salt	Calories: 5, Protein: 0.5g, Carbs: 1g, Fiber: 0.5g	1 cup	0 minutes
Spinach	Low-	Spinach,	Steam or	Calories:	1 cup	5

Food	Description	Ingredients	Instructions	Nutritional Information	Serving Size	Cooking Time
	histamine leafy green	olive oil, garlic, salt	sauté spinach with olive oil and garlic	23, Protein: 2.9g, Carbs: 3.6g, Fiber: 2.2g		minutes
Apple	Low-histamine, nutrient-rich fruit	Apples, cinnamon, honey	Slice and bake apples with cinnamon and honey	Calories: 95, Protein: 0.5g, Carbs: 25g, Fiber: 4.4g	1 medium	20 minutes
Pear	Low-histamine, fiber-rich fruit	Pears, honey, vanilla extract	Slice and roast pears with honey and	Calories: 101, Protein: 0.6g, Carbs:	1 medium	15 minutes

Food	Description	Ingredients	Instructions	Nutritional Information	Serving Size	Cooking Time
			vanilla extract	27g, Fiber: 6g		
Blueberry	Low-histamine, antioxidant-rich berry	Blueberries, lemon juice, honey	Mix blueberries with lemon juice and honey	Calories: 84, Protein: 1.1g, Carbs: 21g, Fiber: 3.6g	1 cup	0 minutes
Peach	Low-histamine, juicy stone fruit	Peaches, honey, cinnamon	Grill peaches and drizzle with honey and cinnamon	Calories: 59, Protein: 1.4g, Carbs: 14g, Fiber: 2.3g	1 medium	5 minutes
Grape	Sweet,	Grapes	Eat	Calories:	1 cup	0

Food	Description	Ingredients	Instructions	Nutritional Information	Serving Size	Cooking Time
	low-histamine fruit		grapes fresh or freeze for a cool treat	62, Protein: 0.6g, Carbs: 15g, Fiber: 0.8g		minutes
Pineapple	Low-histamine, tropical fruit	Pineapple, mint	Dice and mix pineapple with fresh mint	Calories: 82, Protein: 0.9g, Carbs: 21.6g, Fiber: 2.3g	1 cup	0 minutes
Watermelon	Refreshing low-histamine fruit	Watermelon	Slice watermelon and serve	Calories: 46, Protein: 0.9g,	1 cup	0 minutes

Food	Description	Ingredients	Instructions	Nutritional Information	Serving Size	Cooking Time
			chilled	Carbs: 11.5g, Fiber: 0.6g		

Each of these vegetables and fruits offers a nutritious and safe option for those managing histamine intolerance. The simple instructions and minimal cooking times make it easy to integrate these healthy choices into your daily meals.

Safe Beverages and Non-Alcoholic Drinks

When managing histamine intolerance, selecting the right beverages can significantly impact well-being.

Beverage	Ingredients	Instructions	Nutrition	Serving Size	Cooking Time
1. Coconut Water	- 1 cup coconut water	- Serve chilled or over ice	Calories: 46	1 cup	0 minutes
			Fat: 0g, Carbs: 9g, Protein: 1g		
2. Herbal Chamomile Tea	- 1 cup water	- Bring water to a boil, steep chamomile tea bag for 5 mins	Calories: 0	1 cup	5 minutes

Beverage	Ingredients	Instructions	Nutrition	Serving Size	Cooking Time
	- 1 chamomile tea bag		Fat: 0g, Carbs: 0g, Protein: 0g		
3. Fresh Lemonade	- 1 cup water	- Mix ingredients, serve over ice	Calories: 25	1 cup	5 minutes
	- Juice of 1 lemon		Fat: 0g, Carbs: 8g, Protein: 0g		
	- 1 tsp honey				
4. Almond Milk	- 1 cup water	- Blend almonds and water, strain	Calories: 30	1 cup	10 minutes
	- 1/4 cup raw almonds		Fat: 2.5g, Carbs: 1g, Protein: 1g		

Beverage	Ingredients	Instructions	Nutrition	Serving Size	Cooking Time
5. Coconut Milk	- 1 cup water	- Blend shredded coconut and water, strain	Calories: 60		10 minutes
	- 1/2 cup shredded coconut		Fat: 5g, Carbs: 2g, Protein: 1g		
6. Ginger Tea	- 1 cup water	- Boil water with ginger slices for 10 mins	Calories: 5	1 cup	10 minutes
	- 3-4 slices fresh ginger		Fat: 0g, Carbs: 1g, Protein: 0g		
7. Apple Cider Drink	- 1 cup water	- Mix ingredients, serve over ice	Calories: 10	1 cup	1 minute

Beverage	Ingredients	Instructions	Nutrition	Serving Size	Cooking Time
	- 1 tbsp apple cider vinegar		Fat: 0g, Carbs: 2g, Protein: 0g		
8. Pear Smoothie	- 1 cup water	- Blend ingredients until smooth	Calories: 70	1 cup	5 minutes
	- 1 pear		Fat: 0g, Carbs: 18g, Protein: 0g		
	- 1/2 cup plain yogurt				
9. Rice Milk	- 1 cup water	- Blend cooked rice with water, strain	Calories: 40	1 cup	10 minutes
	- 1/4 cup cooked rice		Fat: 0g, Carbs: 8g, Protein:		

Beverage	Ingredients	Instructions	Nutrition	Serving Size	Cooking Time
			1g		
10. Berry Infused Water	- 1 cup water	- Mix ingredients, chill for 1 hour	Calories: 10	1 cup	1 hour
	- 1/4 cup mixed berries		Fat: 0g, Carbs: 2g, Protein: 0g		
11. Peppermint Tea	- 1 cup water	- Bring water to a boil, steep peppermint tea bag for 5 mins	Calories: 0	1 cup	5 minutes
	- 1 peppermint tea bag		Fat: 0g, Carbs: 0g, Protein: 0g		
12. Carrot Juice	- 1 cup carrots	- Juice carrots with	Calories: 40	1 cup	10 minutes

Beverage	Ingredients	Instructions	Nutrition	Serving Size	Cooking Time
		juicer, serve chilled			
	- 1/2 cup water		Fat: 0g, Carbs: 10g, Protein: 1g		
13. Rooibos Tea	- 1 cup water	- Bring water to a boil, steep rooibos tea bag for 5 mins	Calories: 0	1 cup	5 minutes
	- 1 rooibos tea bag		Fat: 0g, Carbs: 0g, Protein: 0g		
14. Cranberry Juice	- 1 cup water	- Blend cranberries with water, strain	Calories: 50	1 cup	10 minutes

Beverage	Ingredients	Instructions	Nutrition	Serving Size	Cooking Time
	- 1/2 cup fresh cranberries		Fat: 0g, Carbs: 13g, Protein: 0g		
15. Cucumber Water	- 1 cup water	- Mix ingredients, chill for 1 hour	Calories: 5	1 cup	1 hour
	- 1/4 cucumber, sliced		Fat: 0g, Carbs: 1g, Protein: 0g		

Each of these beverages aligns with a low-histamine diet and provides a refreshing option for those with histamine intolerance. These drinks offer not only variety but also nutritional benefits, making them excellent choices for managing histamine intolerance effectively.

Snack	Ingredients	Instructions	Nutritional Information	Serving Size	Cooking Time
Apple Slices with Honey	- 1 Apple \n- 1 tsp Honey	1. Slice the apple. \n2. Drizzle honey on top.	95 kcal, 0.3g Fat, 25g Carbs, 0.5g Protein	1 Serving (1 Apple)	5 minutes
Rice Cakes with Almond Butter	- 2 Rice Cakes \n- 2 tbsp Almond Butter	1. Spread almond butter on rice cakes.	200 kcal, 10g Fat, 26g Carbs, 6g Protein	1 Serving (2 Cakes)	2 minutes
Homemade Popcorn	- 2 tbsp Popcorn Kernels \n- 1 tbsp Olive Oil \n- 1/2 tsp Salt	1. Heat oil in pot. \n2. Add kernels and cover. \n3. Pop and season.	150 kcal, 10g Fat, 13g Carbs, 2g Protein	2 Servings	10 minutes

Snack	Ingredients	Instructions	Nutritional Information	Serving Size	Cooking Time
Vegetable Sticks and Hummus	- 1 Carrot \n- 1 Cucumber \n- 1/4 cup Hummus	1. Cut vegetables into sticks. \n2. Serve with hummus.	90 kcal, 4g Fat, 11g Carbs, 3g Protein	1 Serving	5 minutes
Banana Oat Cookies	- 1 Ripe Banana \n- 1 cup Oats \n- 2 tbsp Honey	1. Mash banana. \n2. Mix all ingredients. \n3. Bake at 350°F for 15 min	120 kcal, 2g Fat, 26g Carbs, 2g Protein	6 Cookies	20 minutes
Yogurt with Berries	- 1 cup Greek Yogurt \n- 1/2 cup Berries	1. Mix yogurt and berries.	150 kcal, 0g Fat, 20g Carbs, 15g Protein	1 Serving	2 minutes
Rice	- 5 Rice	1. Spread	110 kcal, 3g	1 Serving	2

Snack	Ingredients	Instructions	Nutritional Information	Serving Size	Cooking Time
Crackers with Cottage Cheese	Crackers \n- 1/4 cup Cottage Cheese	cheese on crackers.	Fat, 15g Carbs, 7g Protein		minutes
Nut Mix	- 1/4 cup Mixed Nuts	1. Combine nuts and serve.	170 kcal, 14g Fat, 6g Carbs, 5g Protein	1 Serving	1 minute
Baked Sweet Potato Chips	- 1 Sweet Potato \n- 1 tbsp Olive Oil \n- 1/2 tsp Salt	1. Slice potato thin. \n2. Bake at 400°F for 15-20 min. \n3. Season.	100 kcal, 4g Fat, 17g Carbs, 1g Protein	2 Servings	25 minutes
Avocado Toast	- 1 slice Bread \n- 1/2	1. Toast bread. \n2. Spread	190 kcal, 9g Fat, 22g Carbs, 3g	1 Serving	5 minutes

Snack	Ingredients	Instructions	Nutritional Information	Serving Size	Cooking Time
	Avocado	avocado.	Protein		
Smoothie	- 1 Banana \n- 1 cup Spinach \n- 1 cup Almond Milk	1. Blend all ingredients.	120 kcal, 2g Fat, 27g Carbs, 2g Protein	1 Serving	3 minutes
Cheese and Crackers	- 5 Crackers \n- 2 oz Cheese	1. Slice cheese and serve on crackers.	200 kcal, 15g Fat, 12g Carbs, 8g Protein	1 Serving	2 minutes
Fresh Fruit Salad	- 1/2 cup Blueberries \n- 1/2 cup Grapes \n- 1 Apple	1. Combine all fruits and serve.	100 kcal, 0g Fat, 26g Carbs, 1g Protein	1 Serving	5 minutes
Rice Pudding	- 1/2 cup Cooked	1. Heat all ingredients	180 kcal, 3g Fat, 33g	1 Serving	10 minutes

Snack	Ingredients	Instructions	Nutritional Information	Serving Size	Cooking Time
	Rice \n- 1 cup Milk \n- 1 tbsp Honey	in saucepan until thickened.	Carbs, 5g Protein		
Coconut Macaroons	- 1 cup Coconut Flakes \n- 1/2 cup Condensed Milk	1. Mix ingredients. \n2. Bake at 350°F for 10 min.	120 kcal, 5g Fat, 20g Carbs, 2g Protein	8 Macaroons	15 minutes

These snacks and foods are easy to prepare, nutritious, and suitable for a low-histamine diet.

Meal Planning and Recipes

21 Days Sample Meal Plans

Day 1

- **Breakfast**: Oatmeal with Fresh Berries
  - Rolled oats cooked with water or almond milk, topped with fresh blueberries and a drizzle of honey.
- **Lunch**: Grilled Chicken Salad
  - Grilled chicken breast served over mixed greens with cucumber, carrots, and olive oil dressing.
- **Dinner**: Baked Salmon with Steamed Vegetables
  - Baked salmon fillet with steamed broccoli and carrots, served with a side of white rice.
- **Snack**: Apple Slices with Peanut Butter

Day 2

- **Breakfast**: Rice Porridge with Fresh Mango
  - Cooked rice mixed with coconut milk and topped with diced mango.
- **Lunch**: Turkey and Avocado Wrap
  - Sliced turkey and avocado wrapped in a lettuce leaf.

- **Dinner**: Stir-Fried Beef with Bell Peppers
  - Stir-fried beef strips with bell peppers and onions, served with brown rice.
- **Snack**: Banana Smoothie

Day 3

- **Breakfast**: Greek Yogurt with Granola
  - Greek yogurt topped with low-histamine granola and sliced strawberries.
- **Lunch**: Quinoa Salad with Grilled Vegetables
  - Cooked quinoa mixed with grilled zucchini, bell peppers, and a light olive oil dressing.
- **Dinner**: Chicken and Vegetable Soup
  - Chicken broth with diced chicken, carrots, celery, and potatoes.
- **Snack**: Rice Cakes with Cottage Cheese

Day 4

- **Breakfast**: Smoothie Bowl
  - Smoothie made with banana, spinach, and almond milk, topped with chia seeds and sliced apple.
- **Lunch**: Tuna Salad Wrap
  - Tuna salad wrapped in a lettuce leaf, served with a side of cucumber slices.
- **Dinner**: Baked Chicken with Sweet Potatoes

- Baked chicken thighs with roasted sweet potatoes and green beans.
- **Snack**: Fresh Fruit Salad

Day 5

- **Breakfast**: Scrambled Eggs with Spinach
    - Scrambled eggs with sautéed spinach, served with a slice of whole grain toast.
- **Lunch**: Grilled Cheese Sandwich
    - Grilled cheese sandwich made with low-histamine cheese and whole grain bread.
- **Dinner**: Baked Cod with Rice
    - Baked cod fillet served with steamed rice and sautéed zucchini.
- **Snack**: Pear with Almond Butter

Day 6

- **Breakfast**: Pancakes with Maple Syrup
    - Pancakes made from gluten-free flour, topped with maple syrup and fresh blueberries.
- **Lunch**: Chicken Caesar Salad
    - Grilled chicken breast on romaine lettuce with olive oil and lemon dressing.
- **Dinner**: Turkey Meatballs with Pasta

- Baked turkey meatballs served with gluten-free pasta and marinara sauce.
- **Snack**: Rice Crackers with Hummus

Day 7

- **Breakfast**: Smoothie with Almond Milk
  - Smoothie made with almond milk, banana, and spinach.
- **Lunch**: Veggie Wrap
  - Wrap with grilled vegetables, lettuce, and olive oil dressing.
- **Dinner**: Lamb Chops with Roasted Potatoes
  - Grilled lamb chops served with roasted potatoes and steamed asparagus.
- **Snack**: Greek Yogurt with Honey

Day 8

- **Breakfast**: Omelette with Mushrooms
  - Omelette filled with sautéed mushrooms, served with a slice of whole grain toast.
- **Lunch**: Shrimp Salad
  - Shrimp salad with mixed greens, cucumber, and olive oil dressing.
- **Dinner**: Baked Chicken with Rice and Beans

- Baked chicken thighs served with white rice and green beans.
- **Snack**: Apple with Peanut Butter

Day 9

- **Breakfast**: Cereal with Almond Milk
    - Gluten-free cereal with almond milk and fresh strawberries.
- **Lunch**: Chicken Stir-Fry
    - Stir-fried chicken with mixed vegetables, served with brown rice.
- **Dinner**: Beef Stew
    - Beef stew with carrots, potatoes, and onions, served with a slice of whole grain bread.
- **Snack**: Rice Cakes with Cottage Cheese

Day 10

- **Breakfast**: Yogurt Parfait
    - Greek yogurt layered with granola and fresh blueberries.
- **Lunch**: Turkey Sandwich
    - Sliced turkey and lettuce on whole grain bread with olive oil spread.
- **Dinner**: Salmon with Quinoa Salad
    - Baked salmon fillet served with a side of quinoa salad.

- **Snack**: Pear with Almond Butter

Day 11

- **Breakfast**: Smoothie with Coconut Milk
    - Smoothie made with coconut milk, banana, and spinach.
- **Lunch**: Veggie Burger
    - Homemade veggie burger served on a gluten-free bun with lettuce and cucumber.
- **Dinner**: Baked Cod with Roasted Vegetables
    - Baked cod fillet served with roasted carrots and potatoes.
- **Snack**: Greek Yogurt with Honey

Day 12

- **Breakfast**: French Toast
    - French toast made with gluten-free bread, topped with maple syrup and fresh strawberries.
- **Lunch**: Chicken Caesar Salad
    - Grilled chicken breast on romaine lettuce with olive oil and lemon dressing.
- **Dinner**: Turkey Meatballs with Spaghetti Squash
    - Baked turkey meatballs served with spaghetti squash and marinara sauce.
- **Snack**: Rice Crackers with Hummus

Day 13

- **Breakfast**: Scrambled Eggs with Tomatoes
  - Scrambled eggs with diced tomatoes, served with a slice of whole grain toast.
- **Lunch**: Tuna Salad Wrap
  - Tuna salad wrapped in a lettuce leaf, served with a side of cucumber slices.
- **Dinner**: Grilled Lamb Chops with Mashed Potatoes
  - Grilled lamb chops served with mashed potatoes and steamed broccoli.
- **Snack**: Fresh Fruit Salad

Day 14

- **Breakfast**: Pancakes with Fresh Fruit
  - Pancakes made from gluten-free flour, topped with sliced bananas and maple syrup.
- **Lunch**: Chicken and Avocado Salad
  - Grilled chicken breast served over mixed greens with sliced avocado and olive oil dressing.
- **Dinner**: Baked Salmon with Couscous
  - Baked salmon fillet served with couscous and roasted vegetables.
- **Snack**: Greek Yogurt with Berries

Day 15

- **Breakfast**: Smoothie with Almond Milk
    - Smoothie made with almond milk, banana, and kale.
- **Lunch**: Quinoa Salad with Grilled Vegetables
    - Cooked quinoa mixed with grilled zucchini, bell peppers, and olive oil dressing.
- **Dinner**: Chicken and Vegetable Soup
    - Chicken broth with diced chicken, carrots, celery, and potatoes.
- **Snack**: Rice Cakes with Cottage Cheese

Day 16

- **Breakfast**: Oatmeal with Honey
    - Rolled oats cooked with water or almond milk, topped with a drizzle of honey.
- **Lunch**: Turkey and Avocado Wrap
    - Sliced turkey and avocado wrapped in a lettuce leaf, served with a side of carrot sticks.
- **Dinner**: Stir-Fried Beef with Broccoli
    - Stir-fried beef strips with broccoli and onions, served with brown rice.
- **Snack**: Banana Smoothie

Day 17

- **Breakfast**: Greek Yogurt with Granola

- Greek yogurt topped with low-histamine granola and sliced apples.
- **Lunch**: Chicken Salad Wrap
    - Chicken salad wrapped in a lettuce leaf, served with a side of sliced cucumber.
- **Dinner**: Baked Chicken with Sweet Potatoes
    - Baked chicken thighs with roasted sweet potatoes and steamed green beans.
- **Snack**: Fresh Fruit Salad

Day 18

- **Breakfast**: Smoothie Bowl
    - Smoothie made with banana, spinach, and almond milk, topped with chia seeds and sliced pear.
- **Lunch**: Shrimp Salad
    - Shrimp salad with mixed greens, cucumber, and olive oil dressing.
- **Dinner**: Baked Cod with Rice
    - Baked cod fillet served with steamed rice and sautéed zucchini.
- **Snack**: Rice Cakes with Peanut Butter

Day 19

- **Breakfast**: Omelette with Spinach

- Omelette filled with sautéed spinach, served with a slice of whole grain toast.
- **Lunch**: Grilled Cheese Sandwich
    - Grilled cheese sandwich made with low-histamine cheese and whole grain bread.
- **Dinner**: Lamb Chops with Roasted Potatoes
    - Grilled lamb chops served with roasted potatoes and steamed asparagus.
- **Snack**: Greek Yogurt with Honey

Day 20

- **Breakfast**: Cereal with Almond Milk
    - Gluten-free cereal with almond milk and fresh strawberries.
- **Lunch**: Chicken Stir-Fry
    - Stir-fried chicken with mixed vegetables, served with brown rice.
- **Dinner**: Beef Stew
    - Beef stew with carrots, potatoes, and onions, served with a slice of whole grain bread.
- **Snack**: Rice Crackers with Cottage Cheese

Day 21

- **Breakfast**: Yogurt Parfait

- Greek yogurt layered with granola and fresh blueberries.
- **Lunch**: Turkey Sandwich
  - Sliced turkey and lettuce on whole grain bread with olive oil spread.
- **Dinner**: Salmon with Quinoa Salad
  - Baked salmon fillet served with a side of quinoa salad.
- **Snack**: Pear with Almond Butter

Lifestyle Adjustments and Coping Strategies

Managing Diet at Home and Socially

Managing histamine intolerance involves lifestyle adjustments that make coping with dietary restrictions at home and socially more manageable. These adjustments center on proactive planning, smart substitutions, and open communication to help individuals navigate their daily lives comfortably while minimizing exposure to histamine-rich foods.

When at home, planning meals is crucial. Creating a weekly meal plan that incorporates low-histamine ingredients can help avoid last-minute decisions that might lead to consuming high-histamine foods. Preparing meals in bulk and freezing individual portions can also prevent food spoilage and reduce histamine buildup, as histamine levels increase in leftovers or stored foods. Keeping a well-stocked pantry with low-histamine staples such as fresh meats, vegetables, and grains ensures that safe meal options are always available.

Substitutions are another key aspect of managing diet at home. Finding alternatives for commonly used high-histamine ingredients can make meals more varied and enjoyable. For example, replacing aged cheeses with fresh cheeses like ricotta or using rice instead of wheat-based products can help maintain a low-histamine diet without sacrificing taste. Exploring new low-histamine recipes and experimenting with different herbs and spices can also keep meals interesting and flavorful.

Dining out can be challenging for those with histamine intolerance, but several strategies can help make the experience more enjoyable. It's important to research restaurants beforehand and choose those with flexible menus or options that can be customized. Calling ahead to inquire about low-histamine choices or to inform the restaurant of dietary needs can also improve the dining experience. When ordering, choosing simple dishes with fresh ingredients and avoiding items that are heavily processed or contain sauces is often a safe bet. Open communication with the waiter and asking for ingredient details can help avoid accidental exposure to high-histamine foods.

Social gatherings and events can be managed by planning ahead. Bringing a low-histamine dish to share or eating a meal beforehand can prevent situations where suitable food options are limited. It's also important to communicate dietary needs to hosts or organizers, who are often understanding and accommodating. Carrying snacks or safe foods when attending events can also provide peace of mind.

In addition to dietary adjustments, lifestyle changes can enhance the management of histamine intolerance. Stress can exacerbate symptoms, so incorporating stress-reducing activities like exercise, meditation, or hobbies can be beneficial. Staying hydrated and avoiding alcohol or beverages that inhibit the DAO enzyme, which helps break down histamine, is also important.

Keeping a food diary to track symptoms and identify potential triggers can be invaluable for managing histamine intolerance both at home and socially. This tool can help individuals become more aware of their unique reactions to different foods and adjust their diets accordingly. It's also a useful resource when consulting healthcare providers for personalized advice or treatment options.

Managing diet at home and socially with histamine intolerance involves a combination of planning, substitutions, communication, and self-awareness. By making these lifestyle adjustments, individuals can enjoy a varied and satisfying diet while minimizing histamine-related symptoms.

Supplements and Medications

Managing histamine intolerance often involves more than just dietary changes, as lifestyle adjustments, supplements, and medications can play crucial roles in alleviating symptoms and improving quality of life.

One of the most widely used supplements for histamine intolerance is diamine oxidase (DAO), which is an enzyme that helps break down histamine in the body. DAO supplements can be particularly useful before meals that might contain high-histamine foods. These supplements are typically taken 15 to 30 minutes before eating and can help mitigate symptoms by enhancing the body's ability to process dietary histamine. DAO supplements are generally well-tolerated and have become a staple for many people managing histamine intolerance.

Another supplement that can be beneficial is vitamin C, which acts as a natural antihistamine by inhibiting histamine release and helping to degrade histamine. Regular intake of vitamin C can assist in reducing histamine levels in the blood, providing relief from symptoms. This supplement can be taken daily as part of a multivitamin or on its own, usually in doses ranging from 500 to 1000 milligrams.

Quercetin is a flavonoid found in various fruits and vegetables that also has antihistamine properties. It stabilizes mast cells, which are involved in histamine release, thereby helping to control symptoms. Quercetin supplements are often taken in doses of 500 milligrams twice daily and can be effective in conjunction with other antihistamine strategies.

Magnesium is another important supplement, as it plays a role in the body's enzyme functions, including those involved in histamine breakdown. Taking magnesium supplements can support overall health and may assist in reducing histamine-related symptoms, with typical doses ranging from 200 to 400 milligrams daily.

Antihistamine medications, both over-the-counter and prescription, are often used to manage histamine intolerance. These medications, such as loratadine, cetirizine, and fexofenadine, block the effects of histamine and provide relief from symptoms like itching, sneezing, and gastrointestinal discomfort. However, they do not address the root cause of histamine intolerance and should be used as part of a broader management strategy.

In addition to supplements and medications, certain probiotics have been found to aid in histamine degradation and gut health, which is crucial for managing histamine intolerance. Strains such as Lactobacillus rhamnosus and Bifidobacterium longum can be beneficial, as they do not produce histamine and may help regulate histamine levels in the gut.

Beyond supplements and medications, lifestyle adjustments like stress management and regular exercise can also help in managing histamine intolerance. Stress is known to exacerbate symptoms, so practices like mindfulness, yoga, and adequate sleep are important for overall well-being and symptom control.

Staying hydrated and avoiding known triggers such as alcohol, smoking, and certain medications can further enhance the effectiveness of these strategies. Additionally, regular consultation with healthcare professionals, such as dietitians and allergists, is essential for personalized advice and effective management of histamine intolerance.

Long-term Management Strategies

Long-term management strategies for histamine intolerance involve a multifaceted approach that encompasses dietary adjustments, lifestyle changes, and coping mechanisms to ensure a better quality of life. These strategies aim to reduce the intake of histamine, manage symptoms, and improve overall wellbeing.

Dietary management is central to controlling histamine intolerance in the long term. A low-histamine diet is essential, which means avoiding foods that are high in histamine or that trigger its release. This includes aged cheeses, cured meats, alcohol, and certain fermented foods. Instead, individuals should focus on fresh, unprocessed foods, such as fresh meats, non-citrus fruits, and most vegetables. Maintaining a food diary can help identify specific triggers and aid in tailoring the diet.

In addition to dietary changes, stress management is crucial, as stress can exacerbate histamine intolerance symptoms. Incorporating relaxation techniques like deep breathing, meditation, or yoga can help manage stress levels. Regular physical activity is also beneficial, as it promotes overall health and can help reduce stress.

Gut health plays a significant role in histamine metabolism. Probiotics and prebiotics can support a healthy gut microbiome, which may help in breaking down histamine more effectively. Regular intake of gut-friendly foods, like yogurt or supplements, can support gut health and reduce symptoms.

For individuals with severe histamine intolerance, enzyme supplementation with diamine oxidase (DAO) can help break down histamine from food, especially when eating out or in situations where dietary control is challenging. However, it's important to use these supplements under medical guidance.

Managing environmental factors is another important aspect of long-term management. Histamine intolerance can be triggered by environmental allergens, so reducing exposure to dust, mold, and pollen can help mitigate symptoms. Using air purifiers, cleaning regularly, and avoiding exposure to known allergens can be beneficial.

Regular medical follow-ups and monitoring are essential for managing histamine intolerance over time. Working with a healthcare provider or dietitian can help individuals stay on track, adjust their diet as needed, and address any emerging symptoms or issues. This professional guidance ensures that the individual's diet remains nutritionally balanced while avoiding high-histamine foods.

Social situations and dining out can pose challenges for those with histamine intolerance. Preparing in advance by researching menus, communicating dietary needs to restaurant staff, or bringing safe snacks can help manage these situations. It's also important to communicate with friends and family about dietary needs to ensure support and understanding.

Mindfulness around food and body awareness are important coping strategies. Being mindful during meals, eating slowly, and paying attention to how different foods affect the body can help manage symptoms and improve digestion. Developing a positive relationship with food, despite dietary restrictions, can also improve overall quality of life.

Overall, long-term management strategies for histamine intolerance require a holistic approach, focusing on diet, lifestyle, and coping mechanisms to maintain health and prevent symptoms.

CONCLUSION

Managing histamine intolerance can be challenging, but with the right guidance and knowledge, it is entirely possible to lead a fulfilling and symptom-free life. The "Histamine Intolerance Food List" offers a comprehensive approach to navigating this condition by providing clear information, practical tips, and delicious recipes tailored to individual needs.

Understanding which foods to avoid and which are safe to consume is crucial for those with histamine intolerance. This guide empowers individuals with the knowledge to make informed decisions, helping to minimize uncomfortable symptoms and improve overall well-being. The carefully curated lists of foods, along with detailed dietary strategies, provide a solid foundation for maintaining a low-histamine diet.

Incorporating a variety of nutrient-rich, low-histamine foods into one's diet not only alleviates symptoms but also promotes better health. The guide's emphasis on freshness, balanced nutrition, and mindful eating helps individuals develop a positive relationship with food, which is essential for long-term success.

For those struggling with histamine intolerance, support is key. The "Histamine Intolerance Food List" addresses this by offering not only dietary advice but also practical tips for managing social situations, handling stress, and maintaining overall gut health. The guide recognizes that each person is unique, and thus provides a flexible framework that can be adapted to individual preferences and lifestyles.

In essence, this guide serves as a valuable resource for anyone dealing with histamine intolerance, offering hope, clarity, and actionable steps for improving health and quality of life. By following the guidance provided, individuals can reclaim their well-being and enjoy a varied and satisfying diet without fear of adverse reactions.